Co|

All rights reserved. No part of this publication maybe reproduced, distributed, or transmitted in any form or by any means, including photocopying, recording, or other electronic or mechanical methods, without the prior written permission of the publisher, except in the case of brief quotations embodied in critical reviews and certain other noncommercial uses permitted by copyright law.

Contents

What Is Chronic kidney disease? 8

Symptoms 9

Stages 12

Treatment 13

    Anemia treatment 14

    Phosphate balance 15

    High blood pressure 15

    Skin itching 15

    Anti-sickness medications 16

    End-stage treatment 16

    Kidney dialysis 17

    Kidney transplant 18

Frequent Causes 19

    Diabetes 20

Hypertension 21

Glomerulonephritis 23

Less Common Causes 24

Risk Factors 26

Diagnosis 29

Complications 31

Prevention 33

Diet 33

The first steps to eating right 35

3-Day Springtime Menu for a Kidney Diet 47

Kidney diet menu: Day 1 47

Kidney diet menu: Day 2 50

Kidney diet menu: Day 3 52

Springtime snack choices 55

CHRONIC KIDNEY DISEASE DIET RECIPES 56

Low Potassium Leached Mashed Potatoes with Roasted Garlic..57

Chicken and Gnocchi Dumplings....................59

Open-Faced Steak & Onion Sandwich Preparation time...62

Turkey & Noodles Preparation time 64

Seafood Croquettes Preparation time 66

Orzo with Tomatoes, Basil, Peas, and Pine Nuts
....68

Chicken 'n' Grape Salad Sandwich 70

Vegan Lettuce Wrap Recipe 72

Veggie Egg 74

Shrimp Salad Preparation time......................77

Crab Cakes 79

Tuna-Noodle Skillet Dinner Preparation time ..80

Chicken Vegetable Salad Preparation time 83

Spicy Lamb Preparation time 84

Stuffed Green Peppers Preparation time 86

Eggplant Casserole Preparation time 88

Fajitas Preparation time 90

Chicken Noodle Soup 92

Herbed Omelet Preparation time 94

French Toast Preparation time....................... 96

Giblet Gravy Preparation time 98

Herb Rice Casserole Preparation time............. 99

Blueberry Muffins Preparation time 101

Rice O'Brien Preparation time...................... 102

Coleslaw Preparation time 104

Fried Onion Rings Preparation time 105

Green Garden Salad Preparation time 107

Baked Egg Custard Preparation time 110

Lemon Crispies Preparation time 112

Jeweled C ookies Preparation time 113

Cream Cheese Cookies Preparation time 115

Pineapple Pound Cake Preparation time 117

Whipped Cream Pound Cake Preparation time 119

Fruit Crunch (Crumb Top Pie) Preparation time 121

Frozen Lemon Dessert Preparation time 122

Fruit Salad Preparation time 124

Chocolate P ie Shell Preparation time 126

Strawberry Sorbet Preparation time 127

Cranberry Punch Preparation time 128

Russian Tea Preparation time 129

Baked Apples with Craisins® Preparation time 130

English Muffin P izza Preparation time 132

What Is Chronic kidney disease?

Chronic kidney disease (CKD) can be a confusing concept to grasp in so far as it is caused by other illnesses or medical conditions. As such, CKD is considered secondary to the primary cause. Moreover, unlike an acute kidney injury (AKI), in which the loss of kidney function may be reversible, CKD is "progressive," which means it gets worse over time. The damage to your kidneys causes scars and is permanent. Among the diseases that can cause CKD are diabetes, hypertension, glomerulonephritis, and polycystic kidney disease.1

Risk factors for chronic kidney disease include older age, low birth weight, obesity, smoking, high blood pressure, diabetes, a family history of kidney disease, and being of African-American descent.

Symptoms

Chronic kidney failure, as opposed to acute kidney failure, is a slow and gradually progressive disease. Even if one kidney stops functioning, the other can carry out normal functions. It is not usually until the disease is fairly well advanced and the condition has become severe that signs and symptoms are noticeable; by which time most of the damage is irreversible.

It is important that people who are at high risk of developing kidney disease have their kidney functions regularly checked. Early detection can significantly help prevent serious kidney damage.

The most common signs and symptoms of chronic kidney disease include:

- anemia

- blood in urine

- dark urine

- decreased mental alertness

- decreased urine output

- edema – swollen feet, hands, and ankles (face if edema is severe)

- fatigue (tiredness)

- hypertension (high blood pressure)

- insomnia

- itchy skin, can become persistent

- loss of appetite

- male inability to get or maintain an erection (erectile dysfunction)

- more frequent urination, especially at night

- muscle cramps

- muscle twitches

- nausea

- pain on the side or mid to lower back

- panting (shortness of breath)

- protein in urine

- sudden change in bodyweight

- unexplained headaches

Stages

Changes in the GFR rate can assess how advanced the kidney disease is. In the UK, and many other countries, kidney disease stages are classified as follows:

Stage 1 – GFR rate is normal. However, evidence of kidney disease has been detected.

Stage 2 – GFR rate is lower than 90 milliliters, and evidence of kidney disease has been detected.

Stage 3 – GFR rate is lower than 60 milliliters, regardless of whether evidence of kidney disease has been detected.

Stage 4 – GRF rate is lower than 30 milliliters, regardless of whether evidence of kidney disease has been detected.

Stage 5 – GFR rate is lower than 15 milliliters. Renal failure has occurred.

The majority of patients with chronic kidney disease rarely progress beyond Stage 2. It is important for kidney disease to be diagnosed and treated early for serious damage to be prevented.

Patients with diabetes should have an annual test, which measures microalbuminuria (small amounts of protein) in urine. This test can detect early diabetic nephropathy (early kidney damage linked to diabetes).

Treatment

There is no current cure for chronic kidney disease. However, some therapies can help control the signs and symptoms, reduce the risk of complications, and slow the progression of the disease.

Patients with chronic kidney disease typically need to take a large number of medications. Treatments include:

Anemia treatment

Hemoglobin is the substance in red blood cells that carries vital oxygen around the body. If hemoglobin levels are low, the patient has anemia.

Some kidney disease patients with anemia will require blood transfusions. A patient with kidney disease will usually have to take iron supplements, either in the form of daily ferrous sulfate tablets, or occasionally in the form of injections.

Phosphate balance

People with kidney disease may not be able to eliminate phosphate from their body properly. Patients will be advised to reduce their nutritional phosphate intake – this usually means reducing consumption of dairy products, red meat, eggs, and fish.

High blood pressure

High blood pressure is a common problem for patients with chronic kidney disease. It is important to bring the blood pressure down to protect the kidneys, and subsequently slow down the progression of the disease.

Skin itching

Antihistamines, such as chlorphenamine, may help alleviate symptoms of itching.

Anti-sickness medications

If toxins build up in the body because the kidneys don't work properly, patients may feel sick (nausea). Medications such as cyclizine or metaclopramide help relieve sickness.

NSAIDs (nonsteroidal anti-inflammatory drugs)

NSAIDs, such as aspirin or ibuprofen should be avoided and only taken if a doctor recommends them.

End-stage treatment

This is when the kidneys are functioning at less than 10-15 percent of normal capacity. Measures used so far – diet, medications, and treatments controlling underlying causes – are no longer enough. The kidneys of patients with end-stage kidney disease cannot keep up with the waste and fluid elimination process on their own – the patient will need dialysis or a kidney transplant in order to survive.

Most doctors will try to delay the need for dialysis or a kidney transplant for as long as possible because they carry the risk of potentially serious complications.

Kidney dialysis

There are two main types of kidney dialysis. Each type also has subtypes. The two main types are:

Hemodialysis: Blood is pumped out of the patient's body and goes through a dialyzer (an artificial kidney). The patient undergoes hemodialysis about three times per week. Each session lasts for at least 3 hours.

Experts now recognize that more frequent sessions result in a better quality of life for the patient, but modern home-use dialysis machines are making this more regular use of hemodialysis possible.

Peritoneal dialysis: The blood is filtered in the patient's own abdomen; in the peritoneal cavity which contains a vast network of tiny blood vessels. A catheter is implanted into the abdomen, into which a dialysis solution is infused and drained out for as long as is necessary to remove waste and excess fluid.

Kidney transplant

The kidney donor and recipient should have the same blood type, cell-surface proteins and antibodies, in order to minimize the risk of rejection of the new kidney. Siblings or very close relatives are usually the best types of donors. If a living donor is not possible, the search will begin for a cadaver donor (dead person).

Frequent Causes

The kidneys are responsible for filtering waste and regulating water and acid levels in the blood. As part of an interrelated system, the kidneys are prone to damage if any disease alters the flow and/or chemistry of blood entering the kidneys or causes direct injury to the kidneys themselves.

Any damage done to the kidneys will cause harm to other organs as waste, acids, and fluids accumulate to dangerous levels. This can intensify the very condition that triggered CKD in the first place.

Diabetes

Diabetic kidney disease develops in approximately 40% of patients who are diabetic and is the leading cause of CKD worldwide.2 Referred to as diabetic nephritis, the condition affects two of every five people with diabetes and is the most common cause of end-stage renal disease (ESRD).

Diabetes is a disease characterized by abnormally high levels of sugar (glucose) in the blood. Elevated blood glucose can cause harm in many parts of the body, but, with the kidneys, it triggers the excessive production of chemicals known as reactive oxygen species (ROS). These are made up of peroxides and other oxidizing compounds.

Over the course of years, exposure to ROS can damage the filters of the kidneys, called glomeruli. When this happens, larger cells that are meant to be filtered can escape and be eliminated from the body in urine. This is the cause of one of the characteristic symptoms of CKD, called proteinuria, in which abnormally high concentrations of protein are found in the urine.

Hypertension

Hypertension is both a cause and consequence of chronic kidney disease.3 It causes kidney (renal) disease by directly damaging nephrons of the kidney (the filtration units comprised of glomeruli and tubules).

In the same way that high blood pressure can cause the hardening of the arteries (atherosclerosis), it can trigger the hardening of the tiny blood vessels that feed the nephrons.

When this happens, less blood is able to reach the kidneys, resulting in fewer functioning nephrons. Moreover, as the damage progresses, the kidneys will be less able to produce a hormone called aldosterone, which regulates blood pressure.

This creates a spiraling effect in which the cycle of hypertension and kidney damage is accelerated, eventually leading to ESRD as more and more blood vessels are damaged and blocked.

Glomerulonephritis

Glomerulonephritis is a group of diseases that cause inflammation of the glomeruli and nephrons.4 Glomerulonephritis usually affects both kidneys and can occur either on its own or as part of another disease.

While it is often difficult to pinpoint what triggered the inflammatory response, the causes can be broadly broken down as follows:

- Focal segmental glomerulosclerosis, a group of diseases that cause the selective scarring of glomeruli

- Autoimmune disorders, which either damage the kidneys directly (IgA nephropathy or granulomatosis with polyangiitis) or trigger whole-body inflammation that indirectly damages the kidneys (such as with lupus)

• Inherited disorders like polycystic kidney disease, which causes the formation of cysts in the kidneys; Alport syndrome, which damages the blood vessels of the kidneys; or Goodpasture syndrome, which damages kidney membranes

In some cases, the cause of glomerulonephritis is never found.

Less Common Causes

Other, less common causes of CKD in adults and children include:

• Heavy metal poisoning, including lead poisoning

- Hemolytic-uremic syndrome, in which ruptured red blood cells block renal filters (occurs exclusively in children)5

- Hepatitis B and hepatitis C, both of which are associated with glomerulonephritis and renal vascular inflammation

- Interstitial nephritis, inflammation of the kidney tubules often related to the long-term use of analgesics or antibiotics

- Pyelonephritis, a bacterial infection of the kidneys

- Prolonged urinary tract obstruction, including an enlarged prostate, kidney stones, and certain cancers

- Recurrent kidney infections

- Reflux nephropathy, the backing-up of urine into the bladder

In addition to known causes, CKD can often be idiopathic, meaning that the cause cannot be found. This is especially true with children. According to a 2015 study published in the Journal of Clinical Investigation, anywhere from 5% to 25% of pediatric ESRD cases will have known cause.

Risk Factors

There are a number of risk factors that can increase your likelihood of developing CKD. Some are non-modifiable, meaning that you cannot change them, while others are ones you can have influence over.

Among the non-modifiable risk factors associated with CKD:

• Genetics: You may be predisposed to CKD insofar as the risk of ESRD is three to nine times greater if you have a family member with ESRD.

• Race: African-Americans are nearly four times as likely to develop ESRD as Caucasian-Americans. Asian-Americans, Hispanic-Americans, and Native Americans are at risk because they are twice as likely to develop diabetes than their white counterparts.

• Age: CKD is more common in people aged 65 years or older (38%) than in people aged 45 to 64 years (13%) or 18 to 44 years (7%).

- Low birth weight, which is associated with impaired kidney development, resulting in fewer and smaller nephrons.

Among the modifiable risks factors associated with CKD:

- Uncontrolled high blood pressure

- Type 1 diabetes with the onset of disease before age 20

- Poor blood glucose control in people with type 1 or 2 diabetes

- Cigarette smoking, which further constricts renal blood vessels

- Obesity, which contributes to hypertension, the risk of diabetes, and the production adipokines—

inflammatory substances that can cause damage renal tissue

In 2016, 726,331 Americans had kidney failure and needed dialysis or a kidney transplant to survive. More than 500,000 of these patients received dialysis, and more than 215,000 people lived with a kidney transplant. While roughly 100,000 Americans are waiting for a kidney transplant, only 21,167 received one in 2018.

Diagnosis

A doctor will check for signs and ask the patient about symptoms. The following tests may also be ordered:

- Blood test – a blood test may be ordered to determine whether waste substances are being adequately filtered out. If levels of urea and creatinine are persistently high, the doctor will most likely diagnose end-stage kidney disease.

• Urine test – a urine test helps find out whether there is either blood or protein in the urine.

• Kidney scans – kidney scans may include a magnetic resonance imaging (MRI) scan, computed tomography (CT) scan, or an ultrasound scan. The aim is to determine whether there are any blockages in the urine flow. These scans can also reveal the size and shape of the kidneys – in advanced stages of kidney disease the kidneys are smaller and have an uneven shape.

• Kidney biopsy – a small sample of kidney tissue is extracted and examined for cell damage. An analysis of kidney tissue makes it easier to make a precise diagnosis of kidney disease.

• Chest X-ray – the aim here is to check for pulmonary edema (fluid retained in the lungs).

• Glomerular filtration rate (GFR) – GFR is a test that measures the glomerular filtration rate – it compares the levels of waste products in the patient's blood and urine. GFR measures how many milliliters of waste the kidneys can filter per minute. The kidneys of healthy individuals can typically filter over 90 ml per minute.

Complications

If the chronic kidney disease progresses to kidney failure, the following complications are possible:

- anemia
- central nervous system damage
- dry skin or skin color changes
- fluid retention
- hyperkalemia, when blood potassium levels rise, possibly resulting in heart damage
- insomnia
- lower sex drive
- male erectile dysfunction
- osteomalacia, when bones become weak and break easily
- pericarditis, when the sac-like membrane around the heart becomes inflamed
- stomach ulcers

- weak immune system

Prevention

Managing the chronic condition

Some conditions increase the risk of chronic kidney disease (such as diabetes). Controlling the condition can significantly reduce the chances of developing kidney failure. Individuals should follow their doctor's instructions, advice, and recommendations.

Diet

CKD differs from an acute kidney injury (AKI) in that the latter is often reversible. With CKD, any damage done to the kidneys will be permanent. When damaged, fluids and waste normally excreted from the body in urine will "back up" and accumulate to increasingly harmful levels. Much of the waste is the result of the normal metabolism of protein.

Because CKD is progressive, immediate dietary changes would be needed to restrict your intake of protein and substances even if have no symptoms. If the disease progresses and kidney function is further impaired, there may be additional restrictions to your diet.

The dietary guidelines would be based on the stage of disease, which ranges from stage 1 for minimal impairment to stage 5 for ESRD. In addition, you would need to achieve your ideal weight while maintaining the recommended daily nutritional goals outlined in the 2015-2020 Dietary Guidelines for Americans.

Eating Right for Chronic Kidney Disease

You may need to change what you eat to manage your chronic kidney disease (CKD). Work with a registered dietitian to develop a meal plan that includes foods that you enjoy eating while maintaining your kidney health.

The steps below will help you eat right as you manage your kidney disease. The first three steps (1-3) are important for all people with kidney disease. The last two steps (4-5) may become important as your kidney function goes down.

The first steps to eating right

Step 1: Choose and prepare foods with less salt and sodium

Why? To help control your blood pressure. Your diet should contain less than 2,300 milligrams of sodium each day.

- Buy fresh food often. Sodium (a part of salt) is added to many prepared or packaged foods you buy at the supermarket or at restaurants.

- Cook foods from scratch instead of eating prepared foods, "fast" foods, frozen dinners, and canned foods that are higher in sodium. When you prepare your own food, you control what goes into it.

- Use spices, herbs, and sodium-free seasonings in place of salt.

- Check for sodium on the Nutrition Facts label of food packages. A Daily Value of 20 percent or more means the food is high in sodium.

- Try lower-sodium versions of frozen dinners and other convenience foods.

- Rinse canned vegetables, beans, meats, and fish with water before eating.

Look for food labels with words like sodium free or salt free; or low, reduced, or no salt or sodium; or unsalted or lightly salted.

Look for sodium on the food label. A food label showing a Percent Daily Value of 5% or less is low sodium. Also look for the amount of saturated and trans fats listed on the label.

Step 2: Eat the right amount and the right types of protein

Why? To help protect your kidneys. When your body uses protein, it produces waste. Your kidneys remove this waste. Eating more protein than you need may make your kidneys work harder.

• Eat small portions of protein foods.

• Protein is found in foods from plants and animals. Most people eat both types of protein. Talk to your dietitian about how to choose the right combination of protein foods for you.

Animal-protein foods:

• Chicken

• Fish

• Meat

• Eggs

• Dairy

A cooked portion of chicken, fish, or meat is about 2 to 3 ounces or about the size of a deck of cards. A portion of dairy foods is ½ cup of milk or yogurt, or one slice of cheese.

Plant-protein foods:

- Beans

- Nuts

- Grains

A portion of cooked beans is about ½ cup, and a portion of nuts is ¼ cup. A portion of bread is a single slice, and a portion of cooked rice or cooked noodles is ½ cup.

Step 3: Choose foods that are healthy for your heart

Why? To help keep fat from building up in your blood vessels, heart, and kidneys.

- Grill, broil, bake, roast, or stir-fry foods, instead of deep frying.

- Cook with nonstick cooking spray or a small amount of olive oil instead of butter.

- Trim fat from meat and remove skin from poultry before eating.

- Try to limit saturated and trans fats. Read the food label.

Heart-healthy foods:

- Lean cuts of meat, such as loin or round

- Poultry without the skin

- Fish

- Beans

- Vegetables

- Fruits

- Low-fat or fat-free milk, yogurt, and cheese

The next steps to eating right

As your kidney function goes down, you may need to eat foods with less phosphorus and potassium. Your health care provider will use lab tests to check phosphorus and potassium levels in your blood, and you can work with your dietitian to adjust your meal plan.

Step 4: Choose foods and drinks with less phosphorus

Why? To help protect your bones and blood vessels. When you have CKD, phosphorus can build up in your blood. Too much phosphorus in your blood pulls calcium from your bones, making your bones thin, weak, and more likely to break. High levels of phosphorus in your blood can also cause itchy skin, and bone and joint pain.

• Many packaged foods have added phosphorus. Look for phosphorus—or for words with "PHOS"—on ingredient labels.

• Deli meats and some fresh meat and poultry can have added phosphorus. Ask the butcher to help you pick fresh meats without added phosphorus.

Foods Lower in Phosphorus

• Fresh fruits and vegetables

• Breads, pasta, rice

- Rice milk (not enriched)

- Corn and rice cereals

- Light-colored sodas/pop, such as lemon-lime or homemade iced tea

Foods Higher in Phosphorus

- Meat, poultry, fish

- Bran cereals and oatmeal

- Dairy foods

- Beans, lentils, nuts

Dark-colored sodas/pop, fruit punch, some bottled or canned iced teas that have added phosphorus

Light-colored sodas/pop, such as lemon-lime or homemade iced tea

Your health care provider may talk to you about taking a phosphate binder with meals to lower the amount of phosphorus in your blood. A phosphate binder is a medicine that acts like a sponge to soak up, or bind, phosphorus while it is in the stomach. Because it is bound, the phosphorus does not get into your blood. Instead, your body removes the phosphorus through your stool.

Step 5: Choose foods with the right amount of potassium

Why? To help your nerves and muscles work the right way. Problems can occur when blood potassium levels are too high or too low. Damaged kidneys allow potassium to build up in your blood, which can cause serious heart problems. Your food and drink choices can help you lower your potassium level, if needed.

- Salt substitutes can be very high in potassium. Read the ingredient label. Check with your provider about using salt substitutes.

- Drain canned fruits and vegetables before eating.

Foods Lower in Potassium

- Apples, peaches

- Carrots, green beans

- White bread and pasta

- White rice

- Rice milk (not enriched)

- Cooked rice and wheat cereals, grits

Apple, grape, or cranberry juice

Foods Higher in Potassium

- Oranges, bananas, and orange juice
- Potatoes, tomatoes
- Brown and wild rice
- Bran cereals
- Dairy foods
- Whole-wheat bread and pasta
  - Beans and nuts

Some medicines also can raise your potassium level. Your health care provider may adjust the medicines you take.

3-Day Springtime Menu for a Kidney Diet

Spring is a season of renewal—so it's time to put away the hearty winter recipes and find new ones that celebrate more sunshine and warmer days to come. The DaVita® dietitian team came up with a fresh three-day menu that helps incorporate all things spring into your meal planning when you're on a kidney diet.

Kidney diet menu: Day 1

Breakfast

- Ziptop Omelet

- English muffin or toasted bread

- Jam or jelly, margarine or butter

- Fresh grapes

- Coffee or tea

- Sweetener or creamer

Lunch

- Blackened shrimp pineapple salad

- Low-sodium crackers or crisp bread

- Lemon cookies

- Lemon-lime soda

Dinner

- Stuffed green peppers

- Dinner rolls

- Margarine or butter

- Stuffed strawberries

- Sparkling water

Day 1 tips:

- Adjust Ziptop Omelet recipe for the number of omelets you plan to serve. You can make extra to refrigerate for an even quicker breakfast the next day. Reheat in the microwave for 20 to 30 seconds.

- Increase shrimp in the salad if you are on a higher protein diet. Use leftover shrimp to make shrimp spread with crackers for a snack.

- Make lemon cookies and serve as dessert at lunch or for an in-between-meals snack.

- Buy grapes to serve at breakfast—they can be used for the second day's salad and for the third day's dinner, dessert or snack.

- Use the extra pineapple as a snack or a dessert if you have leftovers once you make the blackened shrimp pineapple salad.

- Buy enough strawberries for the stuffed strawberries recipe, the second day's pancake recipe and snacks, if desired.

- Leftover stuffed peppers are easy to refrigerate or freeze for a quick lunch or dinner later in the week.

Kidney diet menu: Day 2

Breakfast

- Egg in a Hole

- Homemade Pan Sausage

- Toasted bread

- Jam or jelly, margarine or butter

- Pineapple juice

Lunch

- Tuna veggie salad

- Sliced bread or pita bread

- Lemon cookies

- Home-brewed iced tea with lemon and sweetener

Dinner

- Slow rotisserie-style chicken

- Red wine vinaigrette asparagus

- Pasta tossed in olive oil and garlic

- Chilled or frozen grapes

- Decaffeinated coffee or herb tea

Day 2 tips

- Make a batch of Homemade Pan Sausage and freeze patties on waxed paper and place in a freezer bag. You can prepare individual servings quickly throughout the week.

- Tuna veggie salad calls for steamed vegetables, but you can add uncooked veggies if desired.

- Home-brewed iced tea tastes fresh and is free of phosphate additives compared to some canned or bottled prepared teas.

- Use leftover chicken from dinner for third day's lunch salad.

Kidney diet menu: Day 3

Breakfast

- Cottage cheese pancakes with fresh strawberries
- Whipped topping or syrup
- Scrambled egg or egg whites
- Coffee or tea
- Sweetener or creamer

Lunch

- Lemon curry chicken salad
- Naan (Indian flatbread) or pita bread
- Cranberry juice

Dinner

- Cilantro-lime cod
- Lettuce, cucumber and carrot salad

- Basic salad dressing

- Steamed Rice

- Luscious Lime Dessert

- Lemon-lime soda

Day 3 tips

- Include the eggs if you need a higher protein breakfast. Use low-cholesterol eggs or egg whites only if you are concerned about cholesterol. Egg whites are very low in phosphorus.

- If you have time, make the lemon curry chicken salad the evening before so flavors can blend together.

- Look for fresh cod or any comparable white fish on sale this week. You can also use frozen cod, sole or halibut.

- The basic salad dressing recipe has only one milligram of sodium for two tablespoons, compared to 250 to 400 mg for commercially prepared salad dressing. It will keep for several weeks in the refrigerator.

- To jazz up steamed rice, add your favorite low-sodium herb seasoning blend. Make extra rice for a kidney-friendly fried rice dish later in the week.

Springtime snack choices

When you have a hankering for something in between mealtimes, reach for a healthy and kidney-friendly snack to hold you over.

- Chilled or frozen grapes

- Fiesta Roll-Ups

- Fresh pineapple

- Lemon cookies

- Low-sodium crackers or crisp bread

- Shrimp spread with crackers

- Strawberries

CHRONIC KIDNEY DISEASE DIET RECIPES

In this part are nutritional recipes to restore the health of your kidneys.

Low Potassium Leached Mashed Potatoes with Roasted Garlic

Preparation time

45 minutes

Ingredients

- 2 large potatoes peeled and diced
- 1 head garlic
- 1 Tbsp olive oil
- 1 Tbsp butter
- 1/4 cup milk
- black pepper to taste
- chives for garnish

- parsley for garnish

Instructions

1. Preheat oven to 400 degrees F.

2. Place potato in pot and fill with cool water and bring to a boil.

3. Meanwhile, cut the top of the garlic head so that the cloves are exposed and drizzle with olive oil.

4. Wrap in aluminum foil and place in oven.

5. Roast for 30 minutes, until softened and golden brown.

6. Once the potatoes have come to a boil, pour out the water and add new water to cover the potatoes.

7. Bring to a boil again, then continue to cook until potatoes are soft.

8. Drain completely.

9. Add butter, milk, and desired amount of garlic. I used about half of the head of garlic.

10. Mash the potatoes.

11. Season with pepper to taste.

12. Garnish with chives or parsley.

Chicken and Gnocchi Dumplings

Preparation time

55 minutes

Ingredients

- 2 pounds chicken breast
- 1 pound gnocchi (store bought)
- ¼ cup grape seed or light olive oil
- 1 tablespoon Better Than Bouillon® Chicken Base (low sodium)
- 6 cups reduced-sodium chicken stock
- ½ cup fresh celery, finely diced
- ½ cup fresh onions, finely diced
- ½ cup fresh carrots, finely diced
- ¼ cup fresh parsley, chopped
- 1 teaspoon black pepper
- 1 teaspoon Italian seasoning

Instructions

1. Place stockpot on stove, add oil and set to high heat.

2. Place chicken in hot oil and brown on all sides until golden brown.

3. Add celery, carrots and onions and continue to cook with chicken until translucent. Add chicken stock and let cook on high heat for 20–30 minutes.

4. Reduce heat and add chicken bouillon, black pepper and Italian seasoning; then stir. Add gnocchi and cook for 15 minutes, stirring constantly.

5. Remove from stove, add parsley and serve.

TIP:

- Save extra soup for an easy leftover meal.

- It can be frozen until ready to defrost, heat and serve.

Open-Faced Steak & Onion Sandwich

Preparation time

20 minutes

Ingredients

4 chopped steaks (4-ounces each)

1 tablespoon lemon juice

1 tablespoon italian seasoning

1 tablespoon black pepper

1 tablespoon vegetable oil

1 medium onion, sliced into rings

4 hoagie rolls, sliced

Instructions Combine meat with lemon juice, italian seasoning and black pepper. Heat oil in frying pan over medium heat.   Brown seasoned steaks on both sides until tender.

Remove and drain on paper towels.

Lower heat

Add onion and sauté until onions are tender. Serve open-faced on sliced hoagie roll, topped with onion rings.

Turkey & Nood les Preparation time

25 minutes

Ingredients

- 2 cups dry elbow macaroni
- 1 tablespoon vegetable or olive oil
- 2 pounds fresh lean ground turkey
- ½ cup green onions, chopped
- ½ cup green pepper, chopped
- 1 14-ounce can regular diced tomatoes
- 1 tablespoon italian seasoning
- 1 teaspoon black pepper

Instructions

1. Cook macaroni in medium boiler in 4 cups of boiling water.

2. Allow to boil for 5 minutes or desired tenderness.

3. Drain and set a side. Heat vegetable oil in a large skillet over medium heat.

4. Add ground turkey and cook until done, stirring occasionally.

5. Add onions, green peppers, diced tomatoes, italian seasoning, black pepper and cooked macaroni.

6. Mix well.

7. Cover and let simmer for 5 minutes or until desired.

8. Serve warm.

Seafood Croquettes Preparation time

20 minutes

Ingredients

- 1 can water packed salmon or tuna (14.75-ounce),
- or 1 pound frozen or fresh crab meat.
- 2 egg whites
- ¼ cup chopped onion

- ½ teaspoon black pepper

- ½ cup plain bread crumb or unsalted cracker crumbs

- 1 tablespoon vegetable oil or cooking spray

- 2 tablespoons lemon juice (optional)

- ½ teaspoon ground mustard (crab only)

- ¼ cup regular mayonnaise (tuna and crab only)

Instructions

1. Drain water from canned meat.

2. Combine all ingredients except oil in a medium bowl.

3. Mix well.

4. Form mixture into 8 separate balls, and then flatten to form patties.

5. Heat vegetable oil in skillet.

6. Place patties in hot oil.

7. Brown patties on each side.

8. If cooked in oil, drain patties on paper towel.

Orzo with Tomatoes, Basil, Peas, and Pine Nuts

Preparation time

25 minutes

Ingredients

- 8 ounces orzo, white or whole wheat

- 1 ½ cups cherry tomatoes, sliced in half

- 1 cup green peas

- ½ cup basil, minced

- ½ tsp salt

- ½ tsp black pepper

- 2 Tbs pine nuts, toasted

- ¼ cup balsamic vinegar

- 2 tsp. Dijon mustard

Instructions

1. Cook orzo according to directions on the box.

2. Rinse with cold water and drain.

3. Thaw frozen peas.

4. Toast pine nuts in sauté pan over low heat until slightly brown. (Caution—they burn easily so watch them!)

5. For the balsamic dressing, whisk together the vinegar and Dijon mustard.

6. Mix all ingredients with the orzo and serve.

Chicken 'n' Grape Salad Sandwich

Preparation time

15 minutes

Ingredients

- 1 cup cooked chicken, chopped

- ½ cup celery, diced

- ½ cup green pepper, chopped

- ¼ cup onion, diced

- 1 cup grapes, sliced

- ⅓ cup mayonnaise

Instructions

1. Toss together chicken, celery, green pepper and onion.

2. Add sliced grapes and mayonnaise.

3. Mix gently.

4. Spread chicken 'n' grape blend on bread, roll, tortilla or pita.

5. Add crisp lettuce or other greens.

6. Serve with fresh or canned fruit.

Vegan Lettuce Wrap Recipe

Preparation time

40 minutes

Ingredients

- ¼ cup white rice, dry
- 1 cup cauliflower
- 1 clove of garlic
- 1 teaspoon ginger, fresh
- 2 teaspoons brown sugar
- 2 tablespoons peanut butter
- 1 tablespoon reduced sodium soy sauce

- 1 tablespoon sesame oil

- 2 tablespoons rice vinegar

- ¼ pound (4 ounces) extra firm tofu

- 1 tablespoon canola oil

- ½ cup carrots, shredded or grated

- 4 medium leaves bibb or butter lettuce

Instructions

1. Pre-heat oven to 400F.

2. Cook rice according to package directions, omitting any salt or butter.

3. Chop the cauliflower into very small pieces, to a rice-like consistency.

4. Mince the garlic and ginger.

5. Blend the garlic, ginger, brown sugar, peanut butter, soy sauce, sesame oil, and rice vinegar in a small blender.

6. Set aside.

Veggie Egg

Preparation time

30 minutes

INGREDIENTS

- 4 whole eggs

- 1 c cauliflower

- 3 c fresh spinach

- 1 garlic clove, minced

- 1/4 c bell pepper, chopped

- 1/4 cup onion, chopped

- 1/4 tsp black pepper

- 1 tbsp oil of choice (coconut or avocado oil is good for high heat)

- fresh parsley and spring onion for garnish

- optional tomatoes on side if no potassium restriction

INSTRUCTIONS

1. Beat eggs with pepper until light and fluffy, set aside.

2. Heat oil over medium heat in large skillet.

3. Add onions and peppers to skillet and saute until peppers are translucent and golden.

4. Add garlic, stirring quickly to combine and immediately adding cauliflower and spinach.

5. Saute vegetables, turn heat to medium-low and cover for 5 minutes.

6. Add eggs, stirring to combine with vegetables.

7. When the eggs are cooked thoroughly, top with fresh parsley or spring onions.

8. If no potassium restriction can serve with a side of bright fresh tomatoes topped with cracker black pepper.

9. A touch of feta or a strong sharp cheese would also be delicious with these

Shrimp Salad Preparation time

40 minutes

Ingredients

- 1 pound shrimp, boiled, chopped and deveined

- 1 hard boiled egg, chopped

- 1 tablespoon celery, chopped

- 1 tablespoon green pepper, chopped

- 1 tablespoon onion, chopped

- 2 tablespoons mayonnaise

- 1 teaspoon lemon juice

- ½ teaspoon chili powder

- ⅛ teaspoon Tabasco® or hot sauce
- ½ teaspoon dry mustard
- lettuce, chopped or shredded (optional)

Instructions

1. Combine all ingredients except lettuce in a mixing bowl

2. mix well.

3. Chill in refrigerator for 30 minutes.

4. Serve as a salad over a bed of lettuce, if desired, or serve on a sandwich.

Crab Cakes

Preparation time 20 minutes

Ingredients

- 1 egg (egg substitute or egg white optional)
- ⅓ cup green or red pepper, finely chopped
- ⅓ cup low sodium crackers
- ¼ cup reduced fat mayonnaise
- 1 tablespoon dry mustard
- 1 teaspoon crushed red pepper or black pepper
- 2 tablespoons lemon juice
- 1 teaspoon garlic powder
- 2 tablespoon vegetable oil

Instructions

1. Combine all ingredients.

2. Divide into 6 balls and form patties.

3. Heat vegetable oil in pan at medium heat or oven at 350ºF.

4. Fry patties 4-5 minutes or bake 15 minutes in oven.

5. Serve warm.

Tuna-Nood le Skillet Dinner

Preparation time

Ingredients

- vegetable cooking spray
- 2 tablespoons minced fresh onion
- ⅔ cup water
- ¼ teaspoon curry powder
- ¼ teaspoon black pepper
- 1 10 ¾-ounce can low sodium cream of mushroom soup, undiluted
- 2 cups hot cooked rotini (corkscrew pasta, cooked without salt or fat)
- ½ cup frozen green peas, thawed
- 1 9 ¼-ounce low sodium albacore tuna, with water, drained
- chopped fresh parsley (optional)

Instructions

1. Coat a large non-stick skillet with cooking spray; place over medium heat.

2. Add onion; sauté until tender.

3. Combine water, curry powder, pepper and soup in a bowl; stir well and add to skillet.

4. Add cooked rotini, peas, and tuna; stir well.

5. Cook uncovered, over low heat 10 minutes, stirring occasionally.

6. Sprinkle with parsley, if desired.

Chicken Vegetable Salad Preparation time

10 minutes

Ingredients

- 1 ½ cups cooked chicken, diced
- ½ cup green pepper, finely chopped
- ½ cup celery, finely diced
- ½ cup onions, finely chopped
- 3 tablespoons pimentos, diced
- ½ cup salad dressing or light mayonnaise
- 1 tablespoon lemon juice

Instructions

1. In a large bowl, combine chicken, green pepper, celery, onions and pimentos.

2. In a small bowl, mix mayonnaise and lemon juice.

3. Pour over chicken mixture.

4. Mix well, cover and chill.

5. Serve in a lettuce cups.

Spicy Lamb Preparation time

8 hours 30 minutes

Ingredients

- ¼ cup vegetable oil
- 1 ½ tablespoons garlic powder
- 3 teaspoons dry mustard
- 1 leg of lamb (trimmed for roasting)

Instructions

1. Blend ingredients for marinade: oil, garlic powder and mustard.

2. Coat leg of lamb with marinade; refrigerate 6-8 hours or overnight.

3. Adjust meat on barbecue spit and roast for 30 minutes per pound or until 170ºF on meat thermometer, basting meat continuously with marinade.

Stuffed Green Peppers Preparation time

40 minutes

Ingredients

- 2 tablespoon vegetable oil
- ½ pound ground lean beef, turkey or chicken
- ¼ cup onions, chopped
- ¼ cup celery, chopped
- 2 tablespoons lemon juice
- 1 tablespoon celery seed
- 2 tablespoons italian seasoning

- 1 teaspoon black pepper
- ½ teaspoon sugar
- 1 ½ cups cooked rice
- 6 small green peppers, seeded with tops removed
- paprika

Instructions

1. Preheat oven to 325ºF.

2. Heat oil in saucepan.

3. Add ground meat, onions and celery, cook until meat is browned.

4. Add all ingredients except green peppers and paprika to sauce pan.

5. Stir together, remove from heat.

6. Stuff peppers with mixture.

7. Wrap with foil or place in a dish and cover.

8. Bake for 30 minutes.

9. Remove and sprinkle with paprika.

Eggplant Casserole Preparation time

55 minutes

Ingredients

- 1 large eggplant

- 2 tablespoon vegetable oil

- ½ cup green pepper, chopped

- ½ cup onion, finely chopped
- 1 pound lean ground beef or turkey
- 2 cups plain bread crumbs
- 1 large egg, slightly beaten
- ½ teaspoon red pepper, optional

Instructions

1. Preheat oven to 350°F.

2. Boil eggplant until tender; drain and mash. Heat oil; add green pepper, onion and ground meat.

3. Sauté until cooked.

4. Add eggplant, bread crumbs and egg, mixing well. Add red pepper to taste, if desired.

5. Bake in casserole dish for 30-45 minutes.

6. Serve warm.

Fajitas Preparation time

30 minutes

Ingredients

- 2 tablespoon vegetable oil

- 1 ½ pounds raw chicken strips or beef strips or shrimp (peeled and deveined)

- 2 teaspoon chili powder

- ½ teaspoon cumin

- 2 tablespoon lemon or lime juice

- ¼ green and/or red pepper, sliced lengthwise
- ½ onion white, sliced lengthwise
- ½ teaspoon dry cilantro
- 4 flour tortillas
- vegetable spray

Instructions

1. Preheat oven to 300ºF.

2. Add vegetable oil to non-stick frying pan over medium heat.

3. Add meat, seasonings and lemon/lime juice; cook for 5-10 minutes or until tender. Add pepper and onion to pan and cook 1-2 minutes.

4. Remove from heat; add cilantro.

5. Place tortillas on foil and move to oven.

6. Heat for 10 minutesDivide mixture between tortillas, wrap and serve.

Chicken Noodle Soup

Preparation time

50 minutes

Ingredients

- 1 pound chicken parts 1 teaspoon red pepper

- ¼ cup lemon juice 1 teaspoon caraway seed

- 3 ½ cups water 1 teaspoon oregano

- 1 tablespoon poultry seasoning 1 teaspoon sugar

- 1 teaspoon garlic powder ½ cup celery
- 1 teaspoon onion powder ½ cup green pepper
- 2 tablespoons vegetable oil
- 1 cup egg noodles
- 1 teaspoon black pepper

Instructions

1. Rub chicken parts with lemon juice.

2. In a large pot, combine chicken, water, poultry seasoning, garlic powder, onion powder, vegetable oil, black pepper, red pepper, caraway seed, oregano, and sugar together.

3. Cook 30 minutes or until chicken is tender.

4. Add remaining ingredients and cook for an additional 15 minutes. Serve hot.

Note:

- Soup may require additional water; if so, add water ½ cup at a time.

Herbed Omelet Preparation time

Ingredients

- 1 ½ teaspoons vegetable oil
- 1 tablespoon chopped onion
- 4 eggs
- 2 tablespoons water

- ¼ teaspoon basil
- ⅛ teaspoon tarragon
- ¼ teaspoon parsley (optional)

Instructions

1. Beat eggs; add water and spices.

2. Heat oil in 8" frying pan over medium heat, add onions and sauté.

3. Remove from pan. Pour mixture into heated frying pan over medium heat.

4. As the omelet sets, lift with a spatula to let the uncooked portion of the omelet flow to the bottom.

5. When the omelet is completely set, add the sautéed onion to the top of the omelet and remove from pan to a serving dish.

French Toast Preparation time

20 minutes

Ingredients

- 4 large egg whites, slightly beaten
- ¼ cup 1% milk
- ½ teaspoon cinnamon
- ¼ teaspoon allspice
- 4 slices white bread (may be toasted)
- 1 tablespoon margarine

Instructions

1. Add milk, cinnamon and allspice to egg whites

2. Dip bread into batter one piece at a time.

3. Place on heated grill or in skillet with melted margarine.

4. Turn bread after it is golden brown.

5. Serve hot with syrup (sugar free if diabetic).

Giblet Gravy Preparation time

30 minutes

Ingredients

- 2 cups chicken broth (homemade from boiled chicken)
- 1 tablespoon all-purpose flour
- 1 hard boiled egg, sliced or chopped
- 1-2 poultry liver or giblets, boiled, chopped

Instructions

1. Stir 1 tablespoon of broth with flour until smooth.

2. Add remaining broth and cook over low heat, stirring constantly.

3. Add boiled egg and giblets.

4. Continue to stir until desired thickness (about 5 minutes).

Herb Rice Casserole Preparation time

Ingredients

- 1 cup white rice, uncooked

- 2 cups chicken stock, unsalted

- ¼ cup green bell pepper, chopped

- ½ teaspoon parsley flakes

- 1 tablespoon vegetable oil

- 3 Fresh green onions, chopped

- 1 tablespoon chives

Instructions

1. Preheat oven to 350°F.

2. Combine all ingredients, and place in casserole dish.

3. Bake in covered casserole for 45-50 minutes or until liquid is absorbed.

Blueberry Muffins Preparation time

45 minutes

- Ingredients 1 egg white ¼ cup margarine ½ cup sugar 7 tablespoons water ½ teaspoon vanilla extract

- 1 teaspoon baking powder

- 1 cup all-purpose flour

- 1 cup blueberries, canned and drained or fresh

Instructions

1. Preheat oven to 375ºF.

2. Beat egg white in a small mixing bowl until stiff.

3. Set aside.

4. Cream margarine and sugar together until smooth.

5. Add water and vanilla, mixing thoroughly.

6. Add baking powder and flour.

7. Fold in beaten egg white and blueberries.

8. Bake in greased muffin pan for 30 minutes.

Rice O'Brien Preparation time

20 minutes

Ingredients

- 1½ cup water

- 1 cup rice, uncooked
- ½ cup onion, thinly sliced or chopped
- ¼ cup green pepper, chopped
- ¼ cup carrots, shredded
- ¼ teaspoon red pepper
- ½ teaspoon black pepper
- ½ teaspoon thyme or rosemary
- 1 tablespoon lemon juice
- 1 tablespoon margarine

Instructions

1. In a large saucepan with water boiling, combine all ingredients.

2. Let simmer in covered pan for 15 minutes (do not stir).

3. Remove from pan; fluff rice lightly with fork.

Coleslaw Preparation time

10 minutes

Ingredients

- 1 cup cabbage, shredded

- 2 tablespoons green pepper, chopped

- ¼ cup onion, chopped

- ¼ cup carrots, shredded

- ¼ cup mayonnaise

- 2 tablespoons vinegar

- 1 tablespoon sugar

- ½ teaspoon black pepper

- ½ teaspoon celery seed (optional)
- ⅛ teaspoon dill weeds (optional)

Instructions

1. Combine vegetables.
2. Blend mayonnaise, vinegar and seasonings.
3. Pour over vegetables and toss.

Fried Onion Rings Preparation time

10 minutes

Ingredients

- ¾ cup plain cornmeal
- ¼ cup all-purpose flour

- 1 teaspoon sugar

- 4 medium onions

- 1 egg, beaten

- ¼ cup water

- ½ cup vegetable oil for frying

Instructions

1. Mix cornmeal, flour and sugar together; set aside.

2. Peel onions, and cut crosswise about ¼" thick.

3. Separate into rings.

4. Mix beaten egg and water.

5. Dip rings in egg wash, then into cornmeal mixture.

6. Fry rings for 3-5 minutes in hot vegetable oil, turning until brown.

7. Drain on paper towel. Serve hot.

Green Garden Salad Preparation time

5 minutes

Ingredients

- 4 cups red leaf or other lettuce, shredded
- 1 carrot, sliced
- 2 celery stalks, sliced
- 2 cucumbers, sliced
- 2 radishes, sliced

- 1 large bell pepper, diced or sliced into rings

Instructions

1. Combine vegetables in a large bowl and toss.

2. May serve with your favorite salad dressing.

Spicy Barbecue Sauce Preparation time

15 minutes

Ingredients

- ¼ cup dark corn syrup

- ¼ cup red wine vinegar

- ¼ cup onion, chopped

- 1 cup water

- 2 teaspoons dry mustard

- 2 tablespoons tomato paste

- 1 teaspoon Tabasco® pepper sauce

- 2 tablespoons vegetable oil

- 1 tablespoon all purpose flour

- 1 teaspoon Mrs. Dash® (of your choice)

Instructions

1. Mix all ingredients together except vegetable oil and flour in a sauce pan.

2. Mix vegetable oil and flour together in separate container to make paste.

3. Add to sauce pan, cook on low heat until desired thickness is reached.

4. Pour or brush on baked or grilled meats.

Baked Egg Custard Preparation time

40 minutes

Ingredients

- 2 medium eggs

- ¼ cup 2% milk

- 3 tablespoons sugar

- 1 teaspoon vanilla or lemon extract

- 1 teaspoon nutmeg

Instructions

1. Preheat oven to 325°F.

2. Combine all ingredients, and beat for one minute with electric mixture until thoroughly mixed.

3. Pour into custard cups or muffin pans.

4. Sprinkle nutmeg on top.

5. Bake 20-30 minutes or until knife inserted into the center of the custard comes out clean.

Lemon Crispies Preparation time

25 minutes

Ingredients

- 1 cup unsalted butter or margarine

- 1 cup granulated sugar

- 1 egg

- 1 ½ teaspoons lemon extract

- 1 ½ cup all-purpose flour, sifted

Instructions

1. Preheat oven to 375°F.

2. Cream butter with sugar.

3. Add egg and lemon extract, beat until light and fluffy.

4. Add flour, mix until smooth.

5. Drop batter by level tablespoon onto ungreased cookie sheet, at least 2" apart.

6. Bake for 10 minutes until brown around the edges.

7. Remove from cookie sheet after the cookies have cooled for a minute.

Jeweled C ookies Preparation time

20 minutes

Ingredients

- ½ cup softened unsalted butter or margarine
- 1 cup brown sugar, packed
- 1 medium egg
- ¼ cup milk
- 1 teaspoon vanilla
- 1 ¾ cups all-purpose flour, sifted
- 1 teaspoon baking powder
- 15 large gumdrops, chopped

Instructions

1. Preheat oven to 400°F.

2. Cream butter, sugar and egg thoroughly.

3. Stir in milk and vanilla.

4. Mix flour with baking powder in a separate bowl. Add to above ingredients.

5. Mix in gumdrops and chill dough for at least one hour.

6. Drop dough by tablespoonfuls onto greased cookie sheet.

7. Bake 8-10 minutes until golden brown.

Cream Cheese Cookies Preparation time

1 hour 30 minutes

Ingredients

- 1 cup butter or margarine, softened

- 1 3-ounce package cream cheese, softened
- 1 cup sugar
- 1 egg yolk
- 2 ½ cups all-purpose flour
- 1 teaspoon vanilla extract
- candied cherry halves

Instructions

1. Preheat oven to 325°F.

2. Cream butter and cream cheese; slowly add sugar, beating until fluffy.

3. Beat in egg yolk; add flour and vanilla, mix well.

4. Chill dough at least one hour

5. Shape dough into 1" balls; place on greased cookie sheets. 6. Gently press a cherry half into each cookie. 7. Bake for 12-15 minutes.

Pineapple Pound Cake Preparation time

1 hour 10 minutes

Ingredients for cake

- 3 cups sugar
- 1 ½ cups butter
- 6 whole eggs and 4 egg whites
- 1 teaspoon vanilla extract

- 3 cups all-purpose flour, sifted

- 1 10-ounce can crushed pineapple (drain and reserve juice)

Instructions

1. Preheat oven to 350°F.

2. Beat together sugar and butter until smooth and creamy.

3. Add eggs and egg whites two at a time, mixing after each addition.

4. Add vanilla. Add sifted flour and mix well.

5. Add drained, crushed pineapple. 6. Bake for 45 minutes to 1 hour. 7. In a medium saucepan, mix together ingredients for glaze. Stir frequently. Bring to a boil, until desired

thickness is reached. Pour over top of cake while hot.

Whipped Cream Pound Cake

Preparation time

1 hour 15 minutes

Ingredients

- 2 sticks margarine or butter, softened
- 3 cups sugar
- 6 eggs
- 3 cups cake flour (sift once before measuring)
- ½ pint whipping cream

- 1 teaspoon vanilla flavoring

Instructions

1. Preheat oven to 350°F.

2. Grease and flour tube pan.

3. All ingredients should be at room temperature.

4. Cream margarine and sugar together until fluffy. 5. Add eggs, one at a time, beating after each addition. 6. Gradually add flour and whipping cream, blending between each addition. 7. Beat well for 30 seconds; stir in vanilla flavoring. 8. Pour batter into tube pan; bake for 50-60 minutes.

Fruit Crunch (Crumb Top Pie)

Preparation time

45 minutes

Ingredients

- 4 large tart apples, pared, cored and sliced
- ¾ cup sugar
- ½ cups all-purpose flour, sifted
- ⅓ cup margarine, softened
- ¾ cup rolled oats
- ¾ teaspoon nutmeg

Instructions

1. Preheat oven to 375°F.

2. Place apples in a greased 8" square pan. 3. Combine remaining ingredients in a medium bowl, and spread over fruit. 4. Bake 30-35 minutes or until fruit is tender and lightly browned.

Frozen Lemon Dessert Preparation time

5 hours 30 minutes

Ingredients

4 eggs, separated

⅔ cup sugar

¼ cup lemon juice 1 tablespoon lemon peel, grated

1 cup whipping cream, whipped

2 cups vanilla wafers (about 40), crushed

Instructions

1. Beat egg yolks until very thick.

2. Gradually beat in sugar, beating well after each addition.

3. Add lemon juice and lemon peel; blend well.

4. Cook in double boiler over hot water stirring constantly until thick.

5. Remove from heat and allow to cool.

6. Beat egg whites until stiff peaks form.

7. Fold egg whites into cooled thickened mixture.

8. Fold in whipped cream

9. Spread 1 ½ cups vanilla wafer crumbs in bottom of freezer tray or 10" x 6" x 1 ½" baking dish.

10. Spoon lemon mixture over crumbs.

11. Top with remaining vanilla wafer crumbs.

12. Freeze until firm, several hours or overnight.

Fruit Salad Preparation time

5 minutes

Ingredients

- 2 cups canned fruit cocktail, drained
- 1 cup canned pineapple chunks, drained
- 1 cup whole or sliced strawberries, hulled
- 1 cup apple, peeled, cored and diced
- 1 cup marshmallows
- ½ cup non-dairy whipped topping

Instructions

1. Combine all fruits together.

2. Add marshmallows and whipped topping; mix well.

3. Refrigerate and serve chilled.

Chocolate P ie Shell Preparation time

40 minutes

Ingredients

3 cups cocoa krispies, crushed

½ stick (4 tablespoons) butter

cooking spray Instructions

1. Place crushed cereal and melted butter in a bowl. Stir well.

2. Spray 9" pie pan with cooking spray.

3. Press mixture into pan.

4. Chill at least 30 minutes before filling.

Strawberry Sorbet Preparation time

5 minutes

Ingredients

- ¼ cup sugar
- 1 cup frozen or fresh strawberries, cleaned,
- 1 tablespoon lemon juice
- ¼ cup water
- 1 ¼ cups crushed or cubed ice

Instructions

1. Place ice in a blender.

2. Add all other ingredients, turn speed to crush or liquefy.

Cranberry Punch Preparation time

5 minutes

Ingredients

- 3 quarts cranberry juice

- 3 quarts pineapple juice 1 quart lemonade, frozen, undiluted

- 1 quart water

- 3 28-ounce bottles ginger ale

Instructions

1. Mix all ingredients together.

2. Chill and serve.

Russian Tea Preparation time

5 minutes

Ingredients

- 2 cups Tang ½ cup sugar 1 dry lemonade mix (2 quart size) 1 cup instant tea 1 teaspoon cloves 1 teaspoon cinnamon

Instructions

1. Combine all ingredients.

2. Store in a covered container.

3. To mix: add one tablespoon to 8-ounces hot water.

4. Serve hot.

Baked Apples with Craisins®

Preparation time

1 hour

Ingredients

- 4 apples for baking

- 1 cup apple juice

- ¼ cup brown sugar, packed

- 2 tablespoon Craisins

- red cinnamon candies

Instructions

1. Preheat oven to 375°F.

2. Wash and core the apples. Set aside.

3. Using a square baking pan (9 "x 9" x 1 ¾"), blend the apple juice and brown sugar.

4. Place apples in pan.

5. Fill apple centers with craisins and cinnamon candies.

6. Place pan in the oven. Spoon juice over apples occasionally during baking to glaze the apples and keep them from drying out.

7. Bake 40 to 45 minutes, or until apples are tender when pierced with a fork.

English Muffin P izza Preparation time

15 minutes

Ingredients

- 1 split english muffin
- ¼ cup pizza sauce
- 2 tablespoons shredded mozzarella cheese

Instructions

1. Toast english muffins.
2. Spread pizza sauce evenly on muffin halves.
3. Sprinkle cheese and add toppings.

4. Place the muffin halves on tray and put into toaster oven, set on broil.

5. Broil for about 5 minutes, watching carefully to remove when cheese is golden and melted.

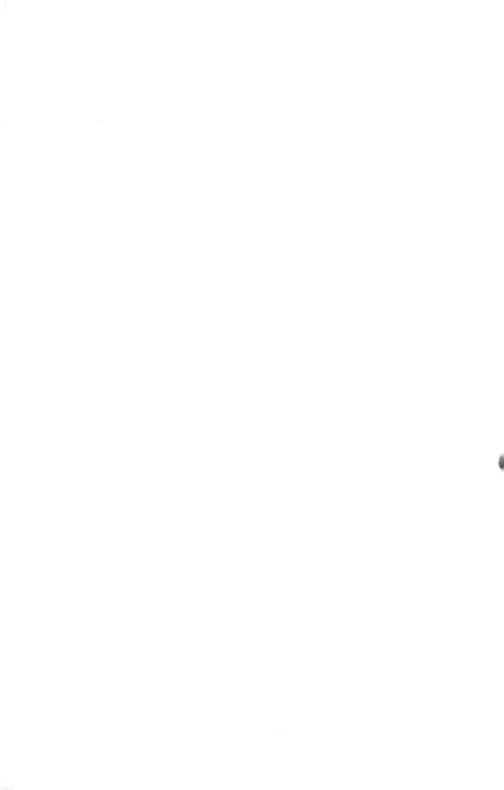